HIROMI KOGA/SACHIYO TARUISHI/NORIKO TSUCHIYA

English for Care and Hospitality I

《ケアとホスピタリティの英語 I》

YUMI PRESS

イラスト・鈴木町子

　　　　　　　　は し が き

　病院の歴史は古い。ということは，病院で働く人々の歴史もそれだけ古いということになる。人類の歴史に病気はつきものであり，現在に至るまで，病気と闘い克服することは，人類の悲願ともいうべき事柄である。病気を治し，癒すことを職務とする医療・看護業務の従事者は，社会から尊敬を受ける機会が多い。尊敬を受けることに甘んじず，患者への尊敬と共に仕事に励む人々は「ケアとホスピタリティの実践者」ということができよう。

　本書は，「ケアとホスピタリティ」をコンセプト（主題）にした総合英語のテキストである。ここでいう「ケア」とは「患者を親身に診て（看て）世話する行為」であり，「ホスピタリティ」とは「患者の身になって接し，心身に快適な環境を提供する行為」である。いずれも，相手を自分の視野に入れて気にかけることからはじまる。そのことを伝えるためには，すぐれたコミュニケーション能力が必要となる。

　社会では，個々人の個性がより際立つ傾向を強め，人間性が問われる機会がますます増えていくであろう。知識や技術は，的確なコミュニケーション能力（ことばとことばによらない表現能力）が発揮されてこそ，より有効に機能するといえる。本書は，高校までの英語力があれば，十分に対応できるテキストであり，医療・看護の現場でケアとホスピタリティあふれる会話ができることを目指した。特徴として，次の項目があげられよう。

　①会話は，平易な言いまわしとし，日本語訳をつけた。
　②「おぼえておきたい phrases, idioms, grammar」は，会話の幅を
　　広げるためのヒントとなる単語，言いまわし，文法をあげた。
　③「EXERCISE」は，聞き取り問題や基本的文法問題など多様な問

題で構成した。
④各ユニットに，ケアとホスピタリティの理解を助けるコラムを入れた。
⑤ Essay1〜5は，トピックスを選んで，日本語訳をつけた。
⑥英語で遊ぶ双六(すごろく)ゲームや，知っておきたい病院内の名称をあげた。
　日本語訳は，あくまで参考とし，自分のことばで考えてみるのもよいであろう。

　本書が，読者の皆さんに少しでも役立つことが出来れば幸いに存じます。最後に，本書の完成に尽力いただいた寺内由美子氏と香坂幸子さんに著者一同，心より感謝申し上げます。

　平成13（2001）年春（新世紀を寿(ことほ)ぎつつ）

著者を代表して　古閑　博美

CONTENTS

はしがき

Unit 1. 朝の挨拶（病室にて）・・・・・・・・・ 2
Unit 2. 検　温 ・・・・・・・・・・・・・・・ 6
Unit 3. 食事のサポート ・・・・・・・・・・・ 10
Unit 4. クスリについて ・・・・・・・・・・・ 14
Unit 5. 検　査 ・・・・・・・・・・・・・・・ 18
Unit 6. 面　会 ・・・・・・・・・・・・・・・ 22
Unit 7. ボランティア ・・・・・・・・・・・・ 26
　　　　USEFUL WORDS ・・・・・・・・・・ 30
Unit 8. 紹介と挨拶 ・・・・・・・・・・・・・ 32
Unit 9. 訪問看護前の打ち合わせ ・・・・・・・ 36
Unit 10. 基本情報 ・・・・・・・・・・・・・・ 40
Unit 11. 生活習慣を聞く ・・・・・・・・・・・ 44
Unit 12. 症状を聞く ・・・・・・・・・・・・・ 48
Unit 13. 生命徴候 ・・・・・・・・・・・・・・ 52
Unit 14. 機能回復訓練 ・・・・・・・・・・・・ 56
Unit 15. 清拭と体位変換 ・・・・・・・・・・・ 60

付録　総復習すごろくゲーム

English for Care and Hospitality I

Unit 1 Morning Greetings

朝の挨拶（病室にて）

DIALOG N=nurse, P=patient

- N: Good morning, Mr. Cox.
- P: Good morning, Ms. Tanaka.
- N: How do you feel today?
- P: About the same.
- N: Oh, could you sleep well last night?
- P: No, I couldn't. It was my first night in the hospital.

　　N＝看護師，P＝患者
- N: おはようございます，コックスさん。
- P: おはようございます，田中さん。
- N: 今日はお加減いかがですか。
- P: 大体同じようです。
- N: あら，ゆうべはよく眠れましたか。
- P: いいえ。病院での最初の夜でしたので。

おぼえておきたい phrases, idioms, grammar

- How do you feel? と同様に使える表現
  How are you?
  How are you feeling today?
  Are you feeling better?
  How are you getting along?
- Replies
  I'm fine, thank you.
  Not very well, I'm afraid.
  I'm a little better, I think.
  I'm feeling much better, thank you.

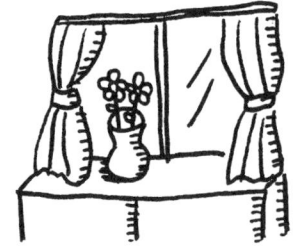

EXERCISE

A．テープを聞いて空所に１語を入れなさい。

P: Good afternoon, Miss Kato.
N: Good afternoon, Mr. Gupta. How are you?
P: Quite (①   ) thank you. (②   ) you?
N: (③   ), thank you.
P: Looks (④   ) rain, doesn't it?
N: It (⑤   ) does.

B．日本文にあうように（　）内に１語を入れなさい。

1. 専門医を紹介しましょう。
   I'll give you the name of a (   ).
2. この用紙に記入してください。
   Please fill out this (   ).
3. どんな症状ですか。
   What (   ) do you have?
4. 太りたいのです。
   I want to gain more (   ).
5. 寝汗をかきます。
   I have night (   ).
6. 眠気を払うことができません。
   I can't shake off this (   ).

C．テープを聞いて書き取りなさい。

1. (7語) _____

2. (6語) _____

D. 次の数字を英語で書きなさい。
1. (TEL) 090-2219-8059 _____
2. $4.40 _____
3. £15.90 _____
4. 100,000 _____
5. 1,000,000 _____
6. 1911年 _____
7. 1/3 _____
8. 2/3 _____
9. 1+3=4 _____
10. 8−2=6 _____
11. 2×4=8 _____
12. 10÷5=2 _____

E. 次の基数詞（Cardinal）を序数詞（Ordinal）に書きかえなさい。
1. one (   )　5. eight (   )
2. two (   )　6. nine   (   )
3. three (   )　7. twelve (   )
4. five (   )　8. twenty (   )

F. 次の数字で示した時間を英語のつづりにしなさい。
1. It is 10 : 00.　It is (   ).
2. It is 2 : 30.　It is (   ) (   ).
3. It is 11 : 57.　It is (   ) (   ).
4. It is 4 : 15.　It is (   ) (   ).
5. It is 5 : 45.　It is (   ) (   ).

G. 次の文の（　）内に入る語を下から選んで書き入れなさい。
　（ただし同じものを２度使ってはいけません）
　1. Mary (　　　) like cats very much.
　2. Tom (　　　) the windows every morning.
　3. There (　　　) many books in this room.
　4. Who (　　　) talking with your mother?
　5. You (　　　) play the piano very well.
　　[aren't, open, can, opens, isn't, doesn't, don't, is]

H. 次の文中の（　）内から正しいものを選びなさい。
　1. This is (egg, an egg, a egg, eggs).　　　(　　　)
　2. These are (pen, a pen, pens, a pens).　　(　　　)
　3. We are (a boy, boys, boy).　　　　　　　(　　　)
　4. He is my (friend, a friend, friends).　　　(　　　)
　5. They aren't (a pupil, pupil, pupils, a pupils). (　　　)

―― Welcome to the hospital. 「ようこそ当院へ」「いらっしゃいませ」――

　ホスピタル (hospital) は,「病院, 動物病院,（品物の）修理店, ホスピタル騎士団の施設」の意味を持つ。古くは,「(老人・孤児・貧困者などを収容した) 慈善施設 (病院, 養老院, 救貧院, 孤児院, 慈善学校など)」を指す語である (『ランダムハウス英和大辞典』第2版)。ラテン語のホスピタリス (hospitalis「もてなしのよい」) の派生語であるホスピターレ (hospitale「中世ラテン語：接待客用宴会場, 後期ラテン語：来客用の部屋」) が, 14世紀に古フランス語で宿泊所や接待所を意味するホスピタルとなり, 16世紀以降「病院」として使用されるようになった。
　今日, 病院に期待されていることはなんであろう。来訪者(患者)に共感し, 好感を与え, 敬意を払うことを具体的に表現することが, 病院でのケア (医療) となりホスピタリティ (看護) となるであろう。ホスピタリティの語源はラテン語の hospes。転じて hospitalis (英語の hospitality) となる。

Unit 2　Take Your Temperature

検温

DIALOG　N＝nurse, P＝patient

N: Mrs. Brown, time to take your temperature. Here's the thermometer.
P: Thank you. I've had no energy since this morning.
N: You must have a fever.
P: I'm afraid I caught a cold.
N: You have a mild fever.
P: Really. I had a chill yesterday.

　　N＝看護師, P＝患者
N: ブラウンさん，検温の時間です。はい体温計です。
P: ありがとう。今日は朝からだるいのです。
N: 熱があるのでは。
P: かぜかもしれないです。
N: 少し熱がありますね。
P: 本当だ。昨日寒気がしていたので。

おぼえておきたい phrases, idioms, grammar

・助動詞 must の用法
　①「〜しなければならない」という当然・義務の意味をあらわす。
　You must start at once.「あなたはすぐ出発しなければなりません」
　②「〜にちがいない」という推断の意味をあらわす。
　It must be true.「それは本当にちがいない」
　　cf. It cannot be true.「それは本当のはずがない」
　③ must の代用 have to〜
　We have to study English.「私たちは英語を学ばなければなりません」

EXERCISE

A． テープを聞いて空所に１語を入れなさい。

N： Mr. White, I will put a (①   ) and a (②   ) on here.

P： Thank you. Please pass me the (③   ).

N： Sorry. I didn't give it to you yet. Here you are.

P： Thank you. By the way, where is my face (④   )?

N： It's on the (⑤   ).

B． 日本文にあうように（ ）内に１語を入れなさい。

1. 体温の記録はつけていますか。
   Are you keeping a (   ) of your (   )?
2. 血圧を計りましょう。
   Let's take your (   ) (   ).
3. あおむけになって身体を楽にしてください。
   Lie on your (   ) and (   ).
4. 下腹部をおさえてください。
   Please press the lower part of your (   ).
5. 医師が私の脈をとりました。
   The doctor took my (   ).

C． テープを聞いて書き取りなさい。

1. (4語) _____

2. (5語) _____

D. テープを聞いて 1～4 の質問に対して正しい答えに○をつけなさい。

1. Which sport is popular in the fall in the United States?
   a. Baseball is.
   b. Baseball and football are.
   c. Football is.
   d. Football and basketball are.
   e. Basketball is.
2. Do most high schools in the United States have football teams?
   a. Yes, they are.
   b. No, they aren't.
   c. Yes, they do.
   d. No, they don't.
   e. They have many teams.
3. When do Americans usually have football games?
   a. They usually have them on Saturday afternoon.
   b. They usually have them on Friday afternoon.
   c. They usually have them on Sunday afternoon.
   d. They usually have them on Saturday morning.
   e. They usually have them on Friday morning.
4. Which sport do Americans enjoy in spring and summer?
   a. They enjoy baseball.
   b. They enjoy football.
   c. They enjoy basketball.
   d. They enjoy winter sports.
   e. They enjoy high school sports.

E． 次の各文を（　）の指示に従って書きかえなさい。
1． That is a white cat.（疑問文）

2． These are animals.（否定文）

3． Mike knows my sister.（疑問文）

4． I can play basketball.（否定文）

F． 次の（　）内に1語を書き入れなさい。
1． We are students.（　　　）school is in the city.
2． Who are those children？（　　　）are my sisters.
3． Look at these pictures. Do you like（　　　）？
4． We have an uncle in London. We love（　　　）very much.

Trust us (me).「信用してください」「おまかせください」「ご心配なく」
　病院で働く人に求められている資質をあげてみたい。
　正直・勤勉・公平・細心・大胆・親切・緻密・正義・明朗・健康・勇気…。なんとも欲張りだが，医療看護の現場では高い技術や最新の知識だけでなく，善き人間的資質が求められている。そして，それらが，さまざまな場面に応じて適切に発揮されることが望まれている。
　大切なのは，"Trust us (me)."とだれに対しても言えるよう精進する（自分を磨く）ことではなかろうか。どんな時でも念入り(check & recheck)に準備し，誠実さを忘れず，相手に真摯に向き合う姿勢を持ちたい。信頼は，相手の目を見て話すことからも生まれる。

Unit 3 Assistance at Mealtime

食事のサポート

DIALOG   N＝nurse, P＝patient

P: I have a burning pain in my throat.
N: You seem to be in pain when you swallow food.
P: Right. But I chew my food well before swallowing it.
N: You had better have jello.
P: I see. I feel feverish.
N: Let me try taking your temperature after you eat.

　　　N＝看護師，P＝患者
P: 喉のあたりが焼けるように痛いのです。
N: 食べ物を飲み込むのが痛そうですね。
P: そうですね。でもよく噛んで飲み込みます。
N: ゼリー類を食べたほうがいいですね。
P: ええ。ちょっと熱っぽいですし。
N: 食後に熱を計ってみましょう。

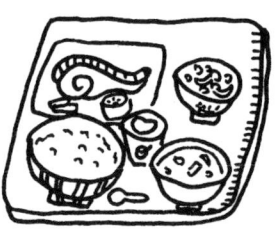

おぼえておきたい phrases, idioms, grammar

・痛さの表現

軽い痛み	mild pain
鈍痛	dull pain
激しい痛み	severe pain, terrible pain, smarting pain
刺す痛み	sharp pain, biting pain
ズキズキの痛み	throbbing pain, shooting pain
	(terrible pain, smarting pain にもこのニュアンスがある)
チクチクの痛み	prickling pain

EXERCISE

A. テープを聞いて空所に1語を入れなさい。

N: It's time for lunch. I have brought your lunch.
P: Oh, it's (①   ) noon?
N: Please make the table (②   ) for lunch.
P: All right. Put it here please.
N: You're having a (③   ) (④   ) today.
P: I know that. I'll have some (⑤   ) food.

B. 日本文にあうように(   )内に1語を入れなさい。

1. 私はカップにお茶をいれた。
   I (   ) tea into my cup.
2. まず箸を持ちます。
   I (   ) (   ) my chopsticks first.
3. 彼女はテーブルをきれいにします。
   She (   ) the table.
4. お碗にラップをかけます。
   You (   ) the bowl with wrap.
5. 彼はお盆を棚に戻します。
   He (   ) the tray (   ) in the cabinet.

C. テープを聞いて書き取りなさい。

1. (5語) _____

2. (9語) _____

D. テープを聞いて空所をうめましょう。

<Essay 1> Global Warming Might Be Boosting Allergies

According to a US Agriculture Department report, (①   ) seems to be raising the levels of allergy-causing ragweed (②   ) in the air.

An American physiologist measured pollen counts on ragweed grown in the (③   ) at various levels of atmospheric CO_2, from the 1900 level of 280 parts per million (ppm) and today's levels of 370 ppm, to the (④   ) predicted level of 600 ppm. Pollen production jumped from 5.5 grams to 10 grams to 20 grams at the three CO_2 levels.

It is said that about one in six Americans suffer from (⑤   ). Common sources of allergy-causing pollens include ragweed, grass, and some trees.

全訳
<エッセイ1>地球温暖化によりアレルギーが増えているかもしれません
　米国農務省の報告によると、地球温暖化により、アレルギーを引き起こす空気中のブタクサ花粉の量が増えているようです。
　あるアメリカの生理学者は、大気中の CO_2（二酸化炭素）のさまざまな濃度のもとに研究所内で育てられたブタクサの花粉の量を測定しました。CO_2 濃度は1900年レベルの280ppm、今日の370ppmから、未来の予測値600ppmまでです。花粉の量はそれぞれ5.5グラムから10グラム、そして20グラムへと大幅に増えました。
　約6人に1人のアメリカ人がアレルギーで苦しんでいると言われています。アレルギーを引き起こす花粉にはブタクサ、草、およびいくつかの木からのものがあります。

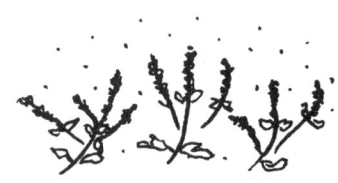

E. 次の文を日本語にしなさい。

High CO_2 levels influenced on our environment and our health.

_____

F. 次の文を英語にしなさい。

1. 花粉の量は二酸化炭素濃度とともに変化します。

_____

2. 世界中でたくさんの人がアレルギーで苦しんでいると言われています。

_____
_____

May I come in？「入ってよろしいですか」「おじゃまします」

　明治期以前の日本家屋は，土・木・紙・竹での建築が一般的であり，家の中は障子や襖（ふすま）で仕切られていた。では，家人のプライバシーはどのようにして保たれていたのであろうか。

　入室に際しては，「お呼びですか」「ただいま参りました」など外から必ず声をかけるのが礼儀であり，中から返事があってはじめて障子（襖）に手をかけ，「御免」「失礼致します」と断って入るのを作法とした。ずかずかと土足で部屋に入るような振る舞いは無作法とされた。一呼吸して相互確認する配慮の文化があった。

　一方，西洋式家屋は石やレンガで造られ，部屋はドアで仕切られている。入室時にはノックする習慣がある。相手の存在を確認する礼儀作法は，造りや方式に関わらずプライバシー尊重や他者配慮に基づく。病院の仕切りはドアやカーテンだが，形態や開閉の状態にかかわらずノック（口ノックもある）し，"May I come in？"と声をかけることを実行しよう。

Unit 4 Asking about Medicine

クスリについて

DIALOG　N＝nurse,　P＝patient

P:　May I ask you a question?
N:　Sure. What's the matter?
P:　Is this medicine very bitter?
N:　Yes, as we say "Good medicine tastes bitter."
P:　That's true, but it's too bad.
N:　After you take the medicine, you should eat some candy.

　N＝看護師，P＝患者
P:　聞いていいですか。
N:　どうぞ。何かあったのですか。
P:　このクスリはとても苦いですか。
N:　ええ，「良薬は口に苦し」と言いますよ。
P:　ええそうですが，でも苦すぎるのもね。
N:　クスリを飲んだ後にキャンディを食べるといいですよ。

おぼえておきたい phrases, idioms, grammar

・ことわざ (proverbs) のいろいろ

The child is the father of the man.	「三つ子の魂百まで」
Easier said than done.	「言うは易く行うは難し」
Like father, like son.	「蛙の子は蛙」
No news is good news.	「便りのないのは良い便り」
Seeing is believing.	「百聞は一見にしかず」
Practice makes perfect.	「習うより慣れよ」
Honesty is the best policy.	「正直は最良の策」
History repeats itself.	「歴史はくり返す」
Health is better than wealth.	「健康は富に勝る」

EXERCISE

A. テープを聞いて空所に1語を入れなさい。

N: This pillbox is (①   ).
P: Really? Do I have to take the medicine in it?
N: Yes. I'll (②   ) how to take the medicine.
P: O.K. I should listen to your advice (③   ).
N: Please take two (④   ) before each meal.
P: I see. Two (⑤   ) before each meal.

B. 日本文にあうように（ ）内に1語を入れなさい。

1. クスリはすぐにききめがあった。
   The medicine had an (   ) effect on me.
2. このクスリを飲めば病気はなおる。
   This medicine will (   ) you of your (   ).
3. 体に注意してもし過ぎることはない。
   You cannot be (   ) careful of your health.
4. 医師は私にたばこを止めるように忠告した。
   The doctor advised me to (   ) (   ) smoking.
5. 処方箋を書きましょう。
   I'll give you a (   ).

C. テープを聞いて書き取りなさい。

1. (7語) _____

2. (9語) _____

D. 次の質問にあなた自身のことについて答えなさい。

1. What is your name?

2. Where do you live?

3. Where were you born?

4. Do you have a cell-phone?

5. What will you do this afternoon?

6. What course are you taking?

7. What time do you get to school?

8. Do you have brothers and sisters?

9. What kind of music do you like?

10. Who is your favorite actor?

11. Can you drive a car?

12. Do you think you'll go to America someday?

E. 次の名詞のうち数えられるものには○, 数えられないものには×を（　）内に書き入れなさい。
1. money（　）　4. milk（　）　7. book（　）
2. butter（　）　5. orange（　）　8. horse（　）
3. chalk（　）　6. table（　）　9. bread（　）

F. 次の各文の（　）内から適語を選び○をつけなさい。
1. He was born (on, at, in) six o'clock (on, at, in) the morning (on, at, in) August 7th (on, at, in) 1980.
2. My aunt started (for, from, at) here (for, from, at) Tokyo last night.
3. (In, On, At) Sunday he does not get up so early. He gets up (at, on, between) seven and eight.

―― Hello.／Good-bye.「こんにちは」「さようなら」 ――

　日本では, 帰宅すると,「ただいま（帰りました）」「お帰り（なさい）」といったやりとりが交わされる。英語では, "I'm home."（ただいま）"Welcome home."（お帰りなさい）"Hello!"（いらっしゃい）"Hi!"（戻ったよ）などと言う。
　他家を訪問したら, "Hello."（ごきげんよう）"How do you do?"（はじめまして）"How are you?"（いかがですか）などの挨拶をする。初めて会う人には必ず自己紹介しよう。
　巡回・訪問介護や看護などでは, 玄関で靴を脱いで奥に入ることになる。靴は爪先を玄関口に向け, 中央でなく, 端によけてそろえよう。コートなどは, 玄関にたたんで置く。じろじろと室内を見回したり, 必要のない場所には立ち入らない。仕事が終わって辞す時は, "Good-bye."(God be with ye (you).「神があなたと共にあられますように」からきたことば) と言うのが, 礼儀正しい。他に, "Take care."（お大事に）"See you soon."（またお邪魔します）など。

Unit 5　Testing

検　査

DIALOG　N＝nurse,　P＝patient

N: Now, it is time for you to go to the testing room.
P: O.K. It's an ECG (electrocardiogram), right?
N: Yes. Turn over on your right side, please. Get up slowly, and you won't feel dizzy.
P: It is hard for me to get out of the bed.
N: Please sit down in this wheel chair. Watch your step.
P: Thank you for your help.

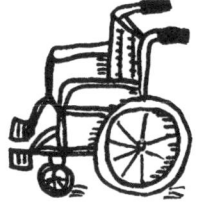

　　N＝看護師，P＝患者
N:　さあ，検査室に行く時間ですよ。
P:　はい，心電図ですね。
N:　そうですよ。右側を下にして横になってください。
　　ゆっくり起きて，そうすれば立ちくらみしません。
P:　ベッドから出るのは大変ですね。
N:　車いすに坐ってください。足もとに気をつけて。
P:　ありがとう。

おぼえておきたい phrases, idioms, grammar

・命令文「～しなさい」，「～して下さい」という文で文頭に動詞の原形がくる。
　Wait a minute.「ちょっと待って」（命令）　Be quiet, please.「どうぞお静かに」（依頼）
・否定の命令文「Don't＋動詞の原形」で「～してはいけない」「～しないで下さい」の意味を表す。
　Don't touch this button.「このボタンに手を触れるな」
・Let's＋動詞の原形　Let us の省略形で「(いっしょに)～しよう」という勧誘の意味を表す。
　Let's go home.「家に帰りましょう」　Let's sing.「歌いましょう」
・命令文＋and「～せよ，そうすれば」命令文＋or「～しなさい，さもないと」の意味を表す。

EXERCISE

A. テープを聞いて空所に1語を入れなさい。

P : Today, I'll take a (①   ).
N : Yes. Please (②   ) on to this stretcher.
P : O.K. (③   ) should I do?
N : Breathe out and (④   ) your whole body, please.
P : But can I take a bath (⑤   ) down?
N : Yes. Now, the bathroom has been (⑥   ).

B. 日本文にあうように（   ）内に1語を入れなさい。

1. 片手がしびれて力が入りにくいようです。
   My hand feels numb and (   ).
2. できるだけリラックスするように。
   Try to relax as much as (   ).
3. 私の検査結果は2日以内で出ます。
   I will receive the test (   ) in two days.
4. 検査のために看護師さんに採血してもらいます。
   I'll have the nurse take a blood (   ) for testing.
5. 何かあったらこのボタンを押して下さい。
   If you need me, just push this (   ).

C. テープを聞いて書き取りなさい。

1. (6語) _____

2. (7語) _____

D. テープを聞いて1〜4の質問に対して正しい答えに○をつけなさい。

1. Is Mr. Tanaka an engineer?
    a. Yes, he does.
    b. No, he isn't.
    c. Yes, he is.
    d. No, he doesn't.
    e. No, he is a pilot.
2. When did Mr. Tanaka go to America?
    a. Eight years ago.
    b. Fifteen years ago.
    c. Nineteen years ago.
    d. Twenty century.
    e. Nineteen eighty-five.
3. How did Mr. Gill come to Japan last month?
    a. He came to Japan by ship.
    b. He came to Japan by train.
    c. He came to Japan by bus.
    d. He came to Japan by car.
    e. He came to Japan by plane.
4. Why was Kyoko very happy at the airport?
    a. Because Mr.Gill spoke to her in Japanese.
    b. Because she wanted to meet Mr. Gill.
    c. Because Daniel spoke to her in Japanese.
    d. Because Mr. Gill came to Japan.
    e. Because she was able to understand what Daniel said in English.

E. 次の日本文にあう英文を①~③の中から選びなさい。

1. テッドとテニスをしたいとき，テッドに
   ① Play tennis, Ted.
   ② Does Ted play tennis?
   ③ Let's play tennis, Ted.

2. お母さんに絵を見てもらいたいとき
   ① There is a picture on the wall.
   ② Does Mother like this picture?
   ③ Look at this picture, Mother.

F. 次の（　）の中に適語を入れなさい。

1. Do you know Mr. Wilson? Yes, I do. I know (　　　) very well.
2. Do you wash your car? Yes, I do. I wash (　　　) car every week.
3. What are these? (　　　) are dictionaries.

―― Take care.「お大事になさってください」「気をつけて」――

　人には，車椅子に乗っていようとベッドに横たわっていようと，あるいはまたいそがしく立ち働いていようと，一つの共通事項がある。それは誰もがこの瞬間，自分のいのちの最先端を生きているという事実である。心して周囲を見回してみよう。かけがえのないいのちが存在し，それぞれの方法や意志を持って自己主張していることの重みが伝わってこよう。

　病院は，医療看護を実施する場所として，社会や人々から必要とされ信頼されている。それにおごることなく，また，裏切ることなく相手に対して敬意を払うことを人間的にも専門的角度からもより深めていきたい。だが，病気や病人に日常的に接することで，逆にそのことに麻痺していく人もいる。一人ひとりに対し，おざなりでなく，いつでも心を込めて，"Take care."と言える人でありたい。それが，いのちの大切さを知る人の態度ではあるまいか。

Unit 6 Visiting

面 会

DIALOG   V=visitor, N=nurse

V: Excuse me, where is Mr. Tada's room?
N: All right. His room is number 315. Turn right, and it's the second room.
V: Thank you. Could you tell me what the visiting hours are?
N: Yes. Visiting hours here are from one to seven.
V: I see. Thank you very much.
N: When you hear music in his room, the time is seven o'clock.
V: Oh, that's a good idea.

V=訪問者，N=看護師
V: おそれいりますが，多田さんの病室はどちらですか。
N: はい。315号室ですよ。そこを右に曲がって，2つめの部屋です。
V: ありがとうございます。面会時間は何時から何時までかを教えていただけませんか。
N: はい。面会時間は1時から7時までです。
V: わかりました。ありがとうございます。
N: 病室に音楽が流れたときが7時ですよ。
V: ええ，それはいいですね。

おぼえておきたい phrases, idioms, grammar

- Where is Mr. Tada's room?と同様に使える表現
  I'm looking for ～. Which way is ～? Could you direct me to ～?
- Replies
  Turn [left / right] [onto / at] ～ street.
  Go straight ahead [for] two blocks.
  Go to the [next light / corner / stop sign].
  Go past ～ on your [left / right].

EXERCISE

A. テープを聞いて空所に１語を入れなさい。

N: This flower (①　　　) was sent to you.
P: I wonder who gave it to me.
N: There is a (②　　　) (③　　　) on it.
P: I can't find it.
N: Here you are. These flowers smell nice and (④　　　).
P: Oh, yes, and what (⑤　　　) flowers!

B. 日本文にあうように（　）内に１語を入れなさい。
 1. 胃の手術をしました。
    I had a (　　　　) operation.
 2. 食餌療法はしていますか。
    Are you on a special (　　　　)?
 3. 腎臓のあたりが痛みます。
    There is a dull pain near my (　　　　).
 4. 医師が痛み止めの注射をしてくれるでしょう。
    A doctor will give me a (　　　　) injection.
 5. この包帯はいつとれるのですか。
    When can I take off this (　　　　)?

C. テープを聞いて書き取りなさい。

 1. (5語) _____

 2. (5語) _____

D. テープを聞いて空所をうめましょう。

<Essay 2> The Avocado Advantage

Avocados are high in fat. So they've earned the (①   ) "butter pear." A medium-sized avocado (②   ) 30 grams of fat. That's why diet experts have long urged Americans to go easy on avocados in favor of less fatty fruits and (③   ). But now nutritionists are taking another look. They're finding that most of the fat in an avocado is monounsaturated, the "good" kind that actually lowers (④   ) levels. Thanks to this new understanding, the U.S. government recently revised its official nutrition guidelines to urge Americans to eat more avocados.

But remember that fat of any type has double the (⑤   ) of the same amount of carbohydrates.

You have to eat them in moderation.

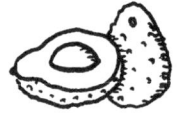

全訳
<エッセイ2>アボカドは健康に良い
　アボカドには脂肪がたくさんあります。それでアボカドに「バター西洋梨」というニックネームがつけられました。中型のアボカドは，30グラムもの脂肪を含んでいます。食餌療法専門家達は，アメリカ人はアボカドを食べるのを減らして，脂肪分がそれほど多くない果実と野菜の方を選ぶよう，長い間勧めてきました。
　しかし，現在，栄養士は別の見解をもっています。彼らは，アボカドの脂肪のほとんどが単一不飽和性，つまりコレステロールレベルを下げる「よい」種類のものであることを知りました。この新しい知識のおかげで，米国政府はアメリカ人に，より多くのアボカドを食べることを勧めようと，最近公式栄養ガイドラインを改訂しました。
　しかし，どのようなタイプの脂肪でも同じ量の炭水化物に比べて2倍のカロリーがあることを覚えておいて下さい。あなたがたは適量食べるようにしなければなりません。

E. 次の文を日本語にしなさい。
That's why diet experts have long recommended Americans to take fruits and vegetables.
___
___

F. 次の文を英語にしなさい。
脂肪はどれだけ多くのカロリーを有していますか。
___

G. 次の（　）の中に適当な英語を記入しなさい。
1. 大－中－小　（　　　　）－（　　　　）－（　　　　）
2. 脂肪　　　　（　　　　）
　　炭水化物　（　　　　）
　　たん白質　（　　　　）
　　ビタミン　（　　　　）

What can I do for you?「私にお申しつけください」「何かお手伝いしましょうか」

　サービス産業は，サービスのあり方として，相手に自分から働きかけることを奨励している。働きかけの行為は，商品や空間の付加価値及び意義を高めるのに貢献するが，接近・接遇術の習得いかんで，相手の反応やその後の人間関係に影響が生じる。
　病院サービスにおいても，人間心理を理解した上で，自分から他者（看護やその家族など）へ積極的に働きかける技術がますます求められている。しかし迫り方によっては，逆に相手の心証を害することになりかねない。TPO (Time, Place, Occasion) に配慮し，笑顔で"What can I do for you?"と声をかけてみよう。
　気遣いを惜しまない人は，病人の心を開き信頼を勝ち取ることができるであろう。あらゆる場面でさりげなくことばをかける訓練を自分に課したい。

Unit 7　Volunteer

ボランティア

DIALOG　N＝nurse,　P＝patient

N: Do you know that a volunteer comes to this ward every Wednesday?
P: No, I didn't know that. How does the volunteer help us?
N: She is a florist, and she takes care of plants and flowers on this floor.
P: Really? She is doing a good thing.
N: If you like, shall I ask her to take care of your flowers?
P: Yes, please.

　N＝看護師，P＝患者
N: 毎週水曜日この病棟にボランティアのかたが来ているのをご存知ですか。
P: いいえ。どんな手助けをしてくださるのですか。
N: 彼女は花屋で、この階の植木や花の手入れをします。
P: そうですか。いいことをなさっていますね。
N: もしよろしければ，あなたのお花の手入れをお願いしましょうか。
P: はい，お願いします。

おぼえておきたい phrases, idioms, grammar

- Do you know ～?　Do you know who he is?「彼が誰だか知っていますか」
  Please tell me who he is.「彼が誰だか教えてください」
- take care of ～　Take care of yourself.「お元気で」
  She will take care of the baby.「彼女は赤ちゃんの世話するだろう」
- If you like ～　You may borrow that book, if you like.
  「もしよろしければこの本を持って行ってもいいですよ」
  If you like, won't you come to my house?「よかったら家にいらっしゃいませんか」

EXERCISE

A． テープを聞いて空所に1語を入れなさい。

V: How are you? May I (①   ) you?
P: Oh, yes. Please come in.
V: There are many flowers in the vase.
P: Yes. I love flowers and my friends give me them as a (②   ).
V: Flowers can (③   ) our heart. I (④   ) you will be fine soon.
P: I hope so. Please change the (⑤   ) of those flowers.

B． 日本文にあうように（　）内に1語を入れなさい。

1. このパジャマを気に入っていただいてうれしい。
   I'm glad that you liked these (   ).
2. 推理小説をお借りできませんか。
   May I borrow your (   ) story novel?
3. このマンガを貸していただけますか。
   Could you lend me this (   ) book?
4. 何か伝言はありますか。
   Do you have some (   )?
5. 病気の話はやめにしましょう。
   Let's quit talking about (   ).

C． テープを聞いて書き取りなさい。

1. (5語) _____

2. (6語) _____

D． 次の動詞の意味を書きそれぞれの活用変化を完成しなさい。

　　　　原形　　　意味　　　過去形　　　過去分詞　　　現在分詞
① take　　（　　　）（　　　）（　　　）（　　　）
②（　　）（　　　）died　（　　　）（　　　）
③（　　）（　　　）（　　　）begun　（　　　）
④（　　）（　　　）（　　　）（　　　）calling
⑤ try　　（　　　）（　　　）（　　　）（　　　）
⑥（　　）（　　　）（　　　）played　（　　　）
⑦（　　）（　　　）hit　（　　　）（　　　）

E． 次の空所をうめなさい。

　　　　原級　　　　比較級　　　　　最上級
① rich　　（　　　　）（　　　　）
② heavy　（　　　　）（　　　　）
③ careful　（　　　　）（　　　　）
④ many　（　　　　）（　　　　）
⑤ famous　（　　　　）（　　　　）
⑥ little　（　　　　）（　　　　）
⑦ thin　（　　　　）（　　　　）

F． 次のAとBの関係とCとDの関係が同じになるようにDに適語を入れなさい。

	A	B	C	D
①	pen	pens	watch	（　　）
②	it	its	they	（　　）
③	America	American	Japan	（　　）
④	boy	boys	lily	（　　）
⑤	this	these	that	（　　）

G．次の文の下線部の語を文の内容に合う語にかえなさい。
1. <u>Summer</u> is a very cold season in Japan.　（　　　）
2. January is the <u>last</u> month of the year.　（　　　）
3. Saturday comes <u>before</u> Friday.　（　　　）
4. Your parents' brother is your <u>aunt</u>.　（　　　）
5. We have <u>lunch</u> in the morning.　（　　　）

H．次の対話文の（　　）内に適する語を下から選んで書き入れなさい。

Tom : I have two rabbits. I like (①　　) very much.
Ken : Do (②　　) have a house?
Tom : Yes, they do. But the house is small. They need a big one.
Ken : (③　　) make a new house for them, Tom.
Tom : Yes, let's. (④　　) to my house on Sunday, Ken.
Ken : All (⑤　　).

[it, they, them, you, do, right, Make, Come, Let's, fast, Okay, Yes, he]

― What's the matter?「どうなさいましたか」「だいじょうぶですか」

　困っている人を見かけたら，その人が知らない人であっても，「どうしましたか」「だいじょうぶですか」などと声をかけるのは，人間として当然の行為として認められよう。しかし果たして，私たちはそうしているであろうか。社会に，「さわらぬ神にたたりなし」といった風潮が蔓延すると，善意を他者に素直に表明できない（しない）人が増えて，よそよそしい関係や空気が広がることになる。
　ホスピタリティとは，相手を自分のことのように気にかけ親切にふるまう行為のことである。病院でホスピタリティを実行するためには，常日頃から観察力を磨き，患者への気配りを徹底する精神（Hospitality Spirit）をやしなう必要がある。自分から"What's the matter?"と声をかけることは，患者への有効な働きかけの第一歩となるであろう。

USEFUL WORDS

Medical Department	Specialist	Affix
Internal Medicine 内科	internist	
Cardiology 循環器科	cardiologist	cardi(o)-心臓, -logy～学
Surgery 外科	surgeon	
Pediatrics 小児科	pediatrician	ped(i)-小児の, -ics～学
Geriatrics 老年病科	geriatrician	ger(i)-老年者
Obstetrics 産科	obstetrician	
Gynecology 婦人科	gynecologist	gyn(e)-女性
Orthopedics 整形外科	orthopedic surgeon	orth(o)-正常な
Dermatology 皮膚科	dermatologist	derm(a)-皮膚の
Urology 泌尿器科	urologist	ur(o)-尿
Ophthalmology 眼科	ophthalmologist	ophthalm(o)-眼
Radiology 放射線科	radiologist	radio-X 線
Psychiatry 精神科	psychiatrist	psych(o)-心
Neurology 神経科	neurologist	neur(o)-神経
Otolaryngology 耳鼻咽喉科	otolaryngologist	ot(o)-耳
ENT(ear, nose & throat)	ENT specialist	laryng(o)-喉頭の

Nurse

director of nursing	看護部長
head nurse	看護師長
registered nurse (RN)	正看護師
nurse midwife	助産師
community health nurse	保健師
visiting nurse	訪問看護師
clinical nurse specialist	専門看護師
licensed practical nurse (LPN)	准看護師
nursing student	看護学生

External Body Parts

head	頭	arm	腕
forehead	額	elbow	肘
eye	眼	wrist	手首
nose	鼻	thumb	親指
mouth	口	finger	手の指
cheek	頬	leg	脚
neck	首	thigh	大腿
shoulder	肩	knee	膝
breast	乳房	calf	ふくらはぎ
chest	胸	shin	向うずね
abdomen	腹	foot	足
back	背中	ankle	足首
lower back	腰	toe	足の指
buttock	臀部	heel	かかと

Internal Body Parts

brain	脳	intestine	腸
throat	咽喉	colon	結腸
pharynx	咽頭	appendix	虫垂
trachea	気管	bladder	膀胱
lung	肺	rectum	直腸
heart	心臓	anus	肛門
liver	肝臓	ovary	卵巣
stomach	胃	uterus	子宮
kidney	腎臓	vagina	膣
gallbladder	胆嚢	muscle	筋肉
spleen	脾臓	bone	骨
pancreas	膵臓	joint	関節
duodenum	十二指腸	rib	肋骨

Unit 8　Introduction

紹介と挨拶

DIALOG　N1＝head nurse, N2＝visiting nurse, P＝patient

N1: How do you feel today, Mr. Davis?
P: Much better, thank you, Wada-san.
N1: Let me introduce Ms. Ikeda. She is going to take care of you after you leave this hospital.
N2: I'm Yasuko Ikeda from Visiting Nurse Station. Nice to meet you, Mr. Davis.
P: Hello, nice to meet you too, Ms. Ikeda.

　N1＝看護師長，N2＝訪問看護師，P＝患者
N1: デイヴィスさん，今日のご気分はいかがですか。
P: ずっとよくなりました，ありがとう，和田さん。
N1: 池田さんをご紹介します。ご退院後のお世話をしてくださる方です。
N2: 訪問看護ステーションの池田泰子です。はじめまして，デイヴィスさん。
P: やー，はじめまして，池田さん。

おぼえておきたい phrases, idioms, grammar

・紹介するとき
　This is my colleague, Prof. Hirai.
　I'd like you to meet my family.
・初対面のあいさつ
　(It's) nice to meet you.
　(I'm) glad to meet you.
　(It's) good to see you.
・初対面後別れるときのあいさつ
　(It's) nice meeting you.
　(It's been) nice seeing you.

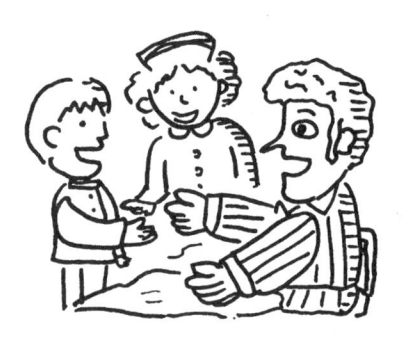

EXERCISE

A．テープを聞いて空所に1語を入れなさい。

N1: How's your mother?
N2: She is doing fine. How's your father doing? Is he (①   )?
N1: Thank you for (②   ). Not so good.
N2: Sorry to (③   ) that. Excuse me. I have to go now. (④   ) you later.
N1: (⑤   ) care. Good-bye.

B．日本文にあうように（　）内に1語を入れなさい。

1. こちらはこの病棟の看護師長の和田さんです。
   (   ) is Ms. Wada, the head nurse of this floor.
2. 同室の方にご紹介しましょう。
   Let me (   ) you to your roommate.
3. はじめまして，よろしく。
   I'm pleased to (   ) you.
4. 具合はよくなられましたか？
   (   ) you feeling better?
5. お会いできてよかったです。
   I enjoyed (   ) you.

C．テープを聞いて書き取りなさい。

1．(4語) _____

2．(5語) _____

D. 次の省略形から，曜日を英語で書きなさい。

Sun. (　　　　)　　Thur. (　　　　)
Mon. (　　　　)　　Fri. (　　　　)
Tue. (　　　　)　　Sat. (　　　　)
Wed. (　　　　)

E. 次の各月の省略形を書きなさい。

January (　　　　)　　July (　　　　)
February (　　　　)　　August (　　　　)
March (　　　　)　　September (　　　　)
April (　　　　)　　October (　　　　)
May (　　　　)　　November (　　　　)
June (　　　　)　　December (　　　　)

F. テープを聞いてそれぞれの患者さんについて書き取りなさい。

PATIENT 1
　Name :
　Address :
　Phone No. :
　Date of birth :

PATIENT 2
　Name :
　Address :
　Phone No. :
　Date of birth :

G. 空所に適切な月を英語で書きなさい。
1. St. Valentine's Day is (　　　　　) 14.
2. Christmas Day is (　　　　　) 25.
3. Girls enjoy the Doll's Festival on (　　　　) 3.
4. Nurses' Day is (　　　　) 12.
5. (　　　　) 31 is Halloween started by the Celts.
6. The Festival of Star Vega is (　　　　) 7.
7. Showa Day is (　　　　) 29.
8. (　　　　) is usually the hottest month in Japan.
9. The 2nd Monday in (　　　　) is Coming of Age Day.
10. Respect for the Aged Day is the 3rd Monday in (　　　　).
11. The rainy season starts toward the end of (　　　　).
12. Labor Thanksgiving Day is (　　　　) 23.
13. My birthday is (　　　　　　).

I'm sorry. 「お気の毒です」「ごめんなさい」「ご愁傷様です」

　マーシャ（Masha）とダーシャ（Dasha）は，1950年1月旧ソビエト連邦のモスクワに生まれた結合性一卵双生児である。特殊な形に生まれたという理由で，生後すぐに親から離され，科学者たちの実験材料となり，研究や論文の対象として扱われた。6才まで，まともな教育も歩き方も学ぶことはなかったという。

　外見の様子から，人から憎まれたり，誤解を受けたりして生きてきた2人だが，「わたしたちがほしかったのは同情ではない。同情されるのと，さげすまれるのとはじつはけっこう近い。そう思うようになった。大人になってから」と言っている（『マーシャとダーシャ』J．バトラー編・武者圭子訳　講談社 2000 p.211）。

　"I'm sorry."ということばに，どれほどの真実が添えられようか。人間理解の奥深さにくじけそうになることもあろうが，ケア（看護）の行為につつしんで取り組みたい。

Unit 9 Arrangements for Visiting

訪問看護前の打ち合わせ

DIALOG   N1=head nurse, N2=visiting nurse,
F=patient's family

N2: When would you like us to come?
F: Let me see. Once a week or twice? What do you think, Wada-san?
N1: Why don't you start with twice?
F: Okay. How about Monday and Thursday afternoon?
N2: Monday and Thursday. Well... at 3 p.m.? Will that suit you?
F: That sounds fine. This Thursday at 3 p.m. at my house, right?

　N1=看護師長，N2=訪問看護師，F=患者の家族
N2: いつ伺うのがよろしいでしょうか。
F: そうですね。週に1度か，2度でしょうかね。和田さんどう思われますか。
N1: まずは週に2度になさったらいかがですか。
F: わかりました。月曜日と木曜日の午後はどうでしょう。
N2: 月曜日と木曜日。えーと，午後3時で，ご都合はいかがですか。
F: けっこうです。今週の木曜日の3時に私の家ですね。

おぼえておきたい phrases, idioms, grammar

・頻度の聞き方と答え方（1）
　How often do you shampoo your hair?
　　Once a day.
　　Twice a week.
　　Three times a month.
　　Four times a year.

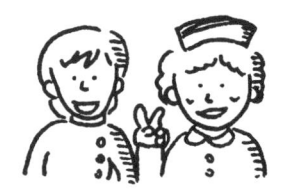

EXERCISE

A. テープを聞いて空所に１語を入れなさい。

N: Dr. Tarle's Office. May I help you?
P: Hello, this is Mrs. Tanaka.
N: Good morning, Mrs. Tanaka. (①   ) can I do for you?
P: My daughter (②   ) a fever of 102 degrees Fahrenheit and a rash on her back.
N: Well, would you like to (③   ) an appointment?
P: Oh, yes, please.
N: Does tomorrow (④   ) at 9:30 suit you?
P: That's fine. (⑤   ) you then.

B. 下の語群から最適な語を選び，空所に書き入れなさい。
1. The nurse (①   ) as a member of a medical (②   ).
2. (③   ) members of the team should consider the (④   ) as the central figure, and should realize that primarily they are all (⑤   ) him.

   | all, patient, team, assisting, works |

C. テープを聞いて書き取りなさい。

1. (9語) _____

2. (9語・2文) _____

D. テープを聞いて空所をうめましょう。

<Essay 3> What Is The Long-term Care Insurance System?
The Nursing Insurance Law was enacted in December 1997, and the Long-term Care Insurance System was implemented in April 2000. This system addresses the issues raised by the rapid growth of the graying population, in particular the care of those who are bedridden or suffering (①　　) senility.
While nursing care for the (②　　) has been provided mainly by the family, people can now (③　　) advantage of comprehensive long-term care services—welfare, health maintenance and medical treatment—provided by this social insurance.
City government, residents and home-nursing assistance firms work together and support each other's efforts at the local level to create a society where residents who need nursing care can live independent lives with dignity. It ensures that (④　　　) who need long-term care and other related services can take optimal (⑤　　　) of what is available based on their own personal rights and choices.

全訳
<エッセイ3>介護保険とは
　平成9年12月に介護保険法が成立し、平成12年4月から制度が開始されました。これは、急速な高齢化で寝たきりや痴呆の高齢者の方々の介護の問題が社会的に大きな課題となっているためです。
　これまでの家族中心による介護から、社会保険方式により、福祉・保健・医療の介護サービスを総合的に受けられるようになります。
　介護等を必要とする区民が、人としての尊厳をもって自立した生活を営む事ができる社会を実現するため、区、区民および事業者の地域社会全体で共同して支えあう仕組みを構築します。介護等を必要とする区民が、自らの権利と選択に基づき、適切な介護サービスを利用できます。
（東京都千代田区のパンフレットから）

E. 左の単語の意味をあらわすものを右から選びなさい。
 1. graying   (　) confined to bed by weakness or old age
 2. bedridden (　) person who live in a place
 3. senility   (　) aging
 4. the elderly (　) weakness of body and mind in old age
 5. resident   (　) rather old people

F. 次の（　）内の語を並べかえて正しい文にしなさい。
 1. 日本では急速な高齢化が進んでいる。
The graying population is (Japan, in, growing, rapidly).

_____

 2. 寝たきりや痴呆の人々も人としての尊厳をもってくらすことができる。
Those who are bedridden or suffering from senility (live, can, dignity, with).

_____

_____

――― Feel free.「お楽（お好き）になさってください」―――

　「あなたは自分の最期をどこで迎えたいですか」と聞かれたら，洋風の生活が増えた今日でも，多くの日本人が，「畳の上（＝自宅）で」と答えるであろう。内心，無理かもしれないと思いながら，人生の終焉を気の休まる馴染みの場所で迎えたいと願うのは，人情というものである。
　自宅で最期を看取ることが容易でなくなった今日，病院で闘病生活を送る人の「快適性・安全性・利便性」や，ホスピス（終末医療機関）の環境整備に配慮と工夫を凝らしたい。すべてにわたって"Feel free."とはいかないであろうが，患者の肉体と精神の解放に少しでも貢献できるよう，尽力したいものだ。

Unit 10　Personal History

基本情報

DIALOG　N=nurse,　P=patient

N: May I ask you some questions about your family?
P: Yes? I have a wife and two sons, aged 30 and 33.
N: Whom do you live with? Are you living alone in Japan?
P: No, I live with my wife. Our children are in the US.
N: Is Mrs. Davis in good health?
P: She sometimes complains of hot flashes due to menopause. Otherwise, she is fit and well.

N=看護師, P=患者
N: ご家族についておたずねしてよろしいですか。
P: なんでしょう。妻と30才と33才になる息子が2人います。
N: どなたとご一緒にお住まいですか。日本では単身でお住まいですか。
P: いや, 妻と一緒です。子供達は米国にいます。
N: 奥様はご健康ですか。
P: 更年期でほてりをうったえることが時々あります。それ以外は元気です。

おぼえておきたい phrases, idioms, grammar

・ていねいな質問の始め方
　May (Can) I ask you some questions?
　I'd (I would) like to ask you a few questions.
・ていねいな質問のしかた
　Could (Would) you tell me your ＿＿＊＿＿?
　　＊full name, current address, permanent address, phone number, date of birth, religion, marital status, occupation

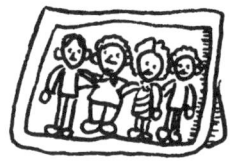

EXERCISE

A. テープを聞いて空所に1語を入れなさい。

A: Hi, I'm Chris from Hong Kong.
B: Hi. My name is Naomi. I'm from Hokkaido.
A: Are you (①   ) the party?
B: Yes, I am. Chris, are you Chinese?
A: No, I'm Chinese Canadian. I'm now (②   ) in a hospital in Hong Kong. Naomi, what do you do?
B: I am a nursing student. I'm (③   ) nursing.
A: How do you like it?
B: We have a (④   ) of work to do. Very busy.
A: Good luck (⑤   ) your nursing study.

B. 右の文が答えとなる質問文を完成させなさい。

1. May I ask how old (   ) (   )?――Twenty years old.
2. (   ) were you born?――I was born in Taipei.
3. (   ) were you born?――I was born on July 2, 1972.
4. (   ) your telephone number?――03-5261-8470.
5. Your (   ), please?――2-3-4, Seijo, Setagayaku.

C. テープを聞いて書き取りなさい。

1. (5語) _____

2. (7語) _____

D. テープを聞き1〜5の場所が下の病院の案内図のどこにあたるのか記号で答えなさい。（毎回病院の入り口からスタートします）

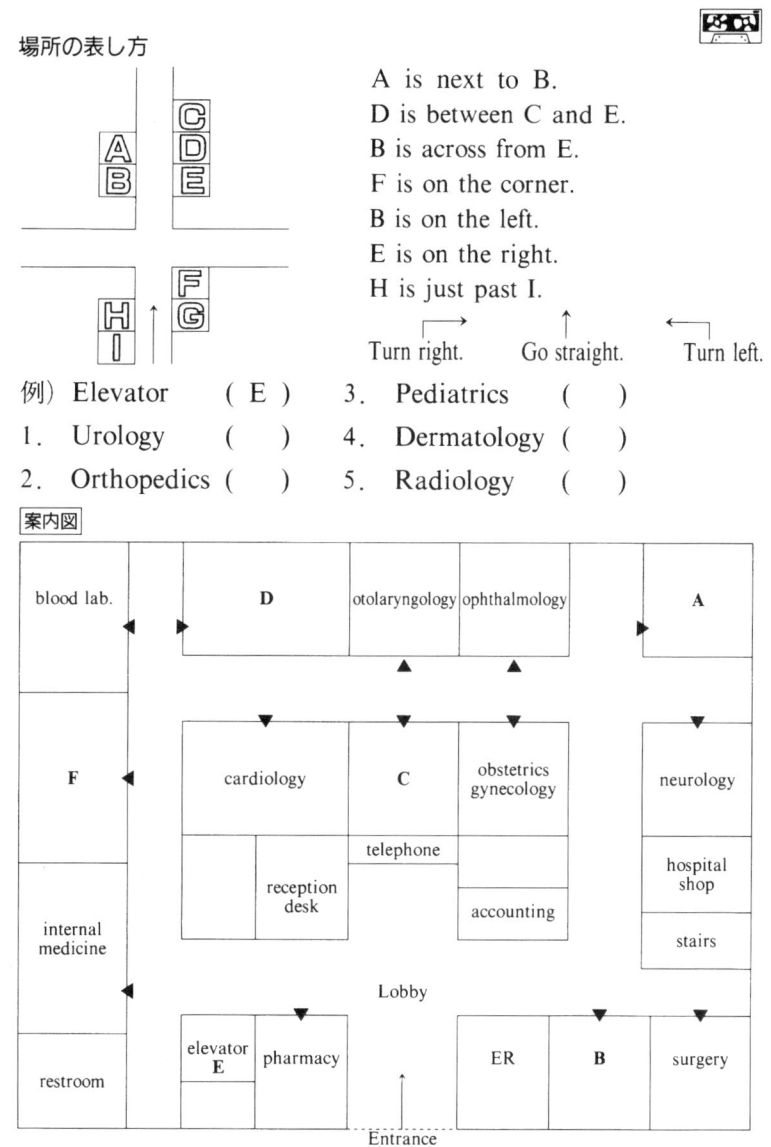

場所の表し方

A is next to B.
D is between C and E.
B is across from E.
F is on the corner.
B is on the left.
E is on the right.
H is just past I.

Turn right.　Go straight.　Turn left.

例）Elevator　　（ E ）　　3．Pediatrics　　（ 　 ）
1．Urology　　（ 　 ）　　4．Dermatology（ 　 ）
2．Orthopedics（ 　 ）　　5．Radiology　　（ 　 ）

案内図

blood lab.	D	otolaryngology	ophthalmology	A
F	cardiology	C	obstetrics gynecology	neurology
		telephone		hospital shop
	reception desk		accounting	
internal medicine				stairs
		Lobby		
restroom	elevator E	pharmacy	ER　　B	surgery

Entrance

E. 単語を並べかえ，日本文の意味になるようにしなさい。
1. お願いがあるのですが。[favor do Would me you a]?

2. はい，何でしょうか。[it , Sure is what]?

3. たばこを吸ってもかまいませんか。
   [mind smoke you I Do if]?

4. 吸わないでいただきたいです。
   [you rather I'd don't].

5. ええ，たばこを吸われてもかまいませんよ。
   [smoke don't I , if mind No you].

Bless you!「お気をつけください」「お大事に」

　風邪を引いたら，くしゃみや鼻水，発熱などいろいろな症状に悩まされることになる。西洋では，くしゃみ (sneezing) は「魂が肉体の外に抜け出る」などとして，不吉の前兆と考えられていた。
　人々は，くしゃみが出たら，神の加護を祈ることや鼻腔を覆い隠すことが有効と考えた。そこで，くしゃみをした人にはすかさず，" (God) bless you!"（「お大事に」）と声をかけ，かけられた人は，"Thank you."と応じるのである。鼻腔を覆うことは，衛生面からも周囲に配慮する有効なポーズといえる。
　"Bless you!"は，感謝やなぐさめの意味を持つことばだが，別れや旅立ちに際しても用いる。"May God bless you!"（「あなたに神のお恵みがありますように」）は，決まり文句としておぼえよう。

Unit 11　Daily Activities

生活習慣を聞く

DIALOG　N=nurse,　P=patient

N: Do you have difficulty sleeping?
P: Hardly ever. I usually sleep well.
N: How's your appetite?
P: Good. I don't have any dietary restrictions now.
N: Nice to hear that. Do you have regular bowel movements?
P: Well, once every three days. I'm often constipated.

　N=看護師，P=患者
N: 眠れなくて困る事がありますか。
P: めったにないですね。いつもよく眠れます。
N: 食欲はいかがですか。
P: ありますよ。今は食事上の制限なしですから。
N: それはよかったですね。便通は規則正しくありますか。
P: そう，3日に1回というところです。便秘がちです。

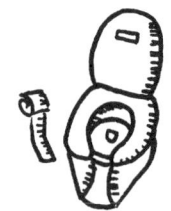

おぼえておきたい phrases, idioms, grammar

(生活習慣は，通例，睡眠と休養，食習慣，排泄，喫煙，飲酒，運動などについてたずねる)

・頻度の表現

　always--- almost always--- often--- sometimes--------------- hardly ever--- never
　100%----------------------------------50%---------------------------------0%

・頻度の聞き方と答え方(2)

　How often do you clean your room?
　everyday / every other day / once every hour / once every two weeks / once every six months

EXERCISE

A. テープを聞いて空所に1語を入れなさい。

N: Tell me (①　　) your eating habits.
P: I (②　　) eat three meals.
N: Do you eat snacks between meals?
P: I (③　　) eat snacks between lunch and (④　　).
N: (⑤　　) your weight!
P: I know.

B. 日本文にあうように（　）内に1語を入れなさい。

1. タバコはお吸いになりますか。
   Do you (　　　)?
2. タバコは1日何箱吸いますか。
   How (　　　) packs of cigarettes do you smoke a day?
3. アルコール類はお飲みになりますか。
   Do you (　　　) alcohol?
4. 1日どれくらいの量を飲みますか。
   How (　　　) do you drink a day?
5. 何か薬を常用していますか。
   Are you (　　　) any medicine regularly?

C. テープを聞いて書き取りなさい。

1. (9語) _____

2. (9語) _____

D. テープを聞いて空所をうめましょう。

<Essay 4> Green Tea May Help Prevent Skin Cancer

It is said that drinking four or more (①   ) of green tea a day may help stave off skin cancer and the substance could be similarly effective if incorporated into skin care creams.

The brew, which is especially popular in Asia, where cancer is rarer (②   ) in the West, contains antioxidants that are known to prevent skin cancer in mice and may prevent it in humans.

Previous research has suggested substances in green tea called polyphenols can kill tumor cells and may starve cancerous growths by limiting (③   ) vessel growth around them.

Based on epidemiological and (④   ) models, we can say drinking four or five cups a day may be very helpful for protection. But it should be (⑤   ) that green tea was a preventive step, not a cure, for skin cancer.

全訳
<エッセイ 4> 緑茶は皮膚癌を防止するのに役立つかもしれない

　1日あたり4杯以上の緑茶を飲むことは皮膚癌をくい止め，またこの物質をスキンケアクリームに混ぜ合わせれば同様な効果がある，と言われています。

　西洋に比して癌が少ないアジアで特によく飲まれているお茶は，マウスの皮膚癌を防止し，人間の皮膚癌も防止するのではないかといわれている抗酸化成分を含んでいます。

　これまでの研究で，ポリフェノールと呼ばれる緑茶の成分が腫瘍細胞を殺すことができて，それらのまわりの血管成長を制限して癌の成長をおさえている可能性を示唆しています。

　疫学とマウスのモデルから，1日あたり4～5杯の緑茶を飲むことは癌の防止に非常に有用であるかもしれないと言うことができます。しかし緑茶は皮膚癌の防止のために役立ちますが，治療のためのものではないことに注意すべきです。

E．次の文を日本語にしなさい。

In addition to drinking four or five cups of green tea a day, eating a lot of vegetables may be very helpful for protection against cancer.

_____

_____

F．次の文を英語にしなさい。

1．あなたは紅茶と緑茶ではどちらが好きですか。

_____

2．緑茶は皮膚癌を防ぐのに役立つかもしれないといわれています。

_____

Zodiac：黄道帯，十二宮

　人体と十二宮の解剖学的対応関係を表わした絵図が残されている。自分の星座はどの部位にあたるのか，興味深い。

　The Ram defends the Head, the Neck the Bull, The Arms, bright Twins, are subject to your Rule; I' th' Shoulders Leo, and the Crab's obeyed I' th' Breast, and in the Guts the modest Maid; I' th' Buttocs Libra, Scorpio warms Desires In Secret Parts, and spreads unruly Fires; The Thighs the Centaur, and the Goat commands The Knees, and binds them up with double bands. The parted Legs in moist Aquarius meet, And Pisces gives Protection to the Feet.（ある古代ローマ時代の詩。17世紀の翻訳。）

　頭－牡羊座，首－牡牛座，腕－双子座，肩－獅子座，胸－蟹座，内臓－乙女座，臀部－天秤座，秘所－蠍座，腿－人馬（射手）座，膝－山羊座，脚－水瓶座，足－魚座。(『イメージシンボル事典』山下主一郎訳他　大修館書店 1984　p.708)

Unit 12　Symptoms

症状を聞く

DIALOG　N＝nurse,　P＝patient

N: What's your problem today?
P: I've been having these headaches for two weeks.
N: How would you describe them?
P: Well, it's a kind of dull pain.
N: Where is the pain? Can you show me?
P: In the front, here. (Pointing his forehead)
N: How long do these headaches last?
P: Sometimes ten minutes, sometimes an hour.

　　N＝看護師，P＝患者
N: 今日はどうなさいましたか。
P: 頭痛が2週間続いていまして。
N: どんな風な頭痛なのかおしゃっていただけますか。
P: そう，鈍痛のような痛みです。
N: 痛みはどのあたりですか。さし示してください。
P: 前のほうのここです。（額を指さして）
N: 頭痛はどれくらいの間続くのですか。
P: 10分の時もあるし，1時間の時もあります。

おぼえておきたい phrases, idioms, grammar

・痛みの表現

　pain（一般的な痛み），ache（通例，身体の一部に継続的に感じる鈍痛），sore（けが，炎症，使い過ぎなどによる痛み），stiff（筋肉等がこった痛み）
　「頭が痛いです」My head aches.　I have a headache.　I have / feel a pain in my head.　My head hurts.

EXERCISE

A． テープを聞いて空所に1語を入れなさい。

D: Do you have a (①   ) or any phlegm?
P: I sometimes cough during the (②   ).
D: Do you perspire while sleeping?
P: Yes. I (③   ) break out in a sweat.
D: How about your energy?
P: (④   ). I feel sluggish these days.
D: How about your (⑤   )? Is it steady?
P: I lost 2 pounds recently.

B． 日本文にあうように（　）内に1語を入れなさい。

1. 痛みますか。　はい，ひどい痛みがあります。
   Do you have (   )? ──── Yes, I have a severe one.
2. どこが痛みますか。　おなかのこのあたり。
   (   ) the pain? ──── Here, in my abdomen.
3. どんな痛みですか。　ずきずきするような痛みです。
   What (   ) of pain is it? ──── It's a throbbing pain.
4. どれくらい続いていますか。　2日間。
   How (   ) have you had the pain? ──── For two days.
5. 何か他の症状はありますか。　寒気と吐き気もします。
   Any other (   )? ──── I feel cold and nauseated.

C． テープを聞いて書き取りなさい。

1. (6語) _____

2. (8語) _____

D. 次の状態のときはどの診療科にいったらよいでしょう。下のクロスワードに書き込みましょう。

ACROSS
① My eye is red and itchy.
② I'm going to have my baby in September.
③ I have a stomachache and diarrhea.
④ I have lower back pain.
⑤ I have a heart trouble.
⑥ I have trouble with my *bladder.
⑦ I have a throbbing toothache.
　　　　　　　　　　　　　　*bladder＝膀胱

DOWN
⑧ My baby has a fever.
⑨ I have trouble with my skin.
⑩ I have a *pollen allergy.　　*pollen＝花粉

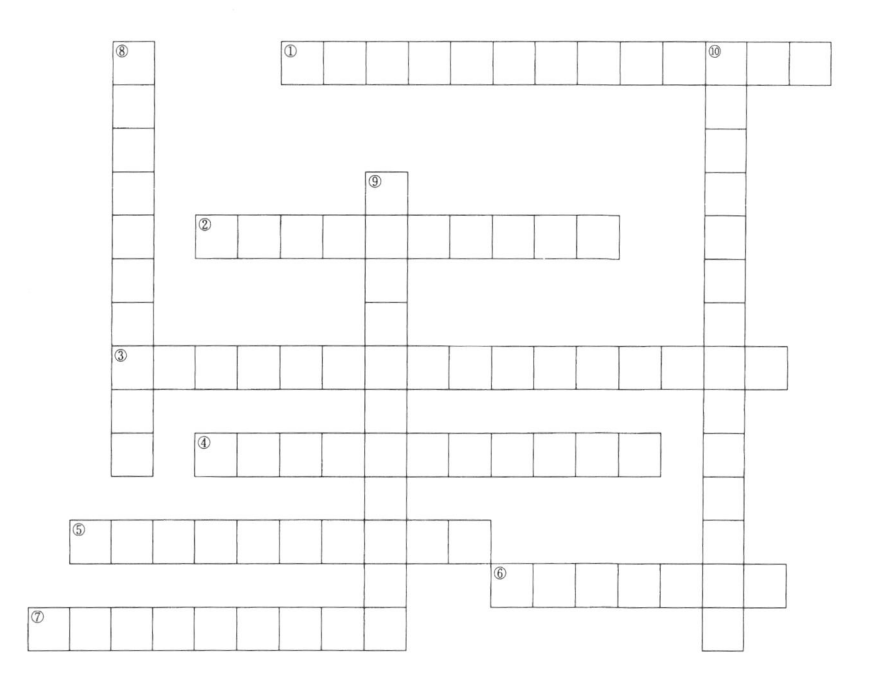

E. 空所に for または since を書き入れなさい。

How long.......?
1. The Parks have lived in Osaka (　　) six years.
2. They have been in their current address (　　) 1994.
3. Mr. Park has been in Seoul (　　) last Friday.
4. Spot has been with the Parks (　　) he was a puppy.
5. Their son has been taking piano lessons (　　) eight years.

F. 左側の文頭と右側の文末を結んで文を完成させなさい。
1. How long have you had　　(　　) describe the pain?
2. Have you had any　　(　　) to any medicine?
3. Are you allergic　　(　　) urinating?
4. Do you have difficulty　　(　　) serious illnesses?
5. How would you　　(　　) these symptoms?

Would you care for smile?「笑顔はお好きですか」「ほほえみはいかがですか」

　ファスト・フードの店頭では，商品だけでなく笑顔も売っている（ことになっている）。ただし，「無料」。笑顔というおまけに出会って，客の気分がわるかろうはずはない。笑顔はまさに，値千金である。笑顔の価値を知る職場やそこで働くこと，あるいは笑顔を絶やさない人々と共に働くことは，そうでない職場や仲間と働く数倍，勤労意識が高まるという。アドレナリンが活発に身体を駆け巡ることで，幸せな人生時間を過ごすことができるだろう。
　病人だって，笑顔に出会いたい。ならば，言われる前や思われる前に，"Would you care for smile?"と先制攻撃してみよう（ことばでなく笑顔それ自体で示すのも有効）。患者の精神は安定し，病気の進行を多少なりとも押しとどめることになる（と信じて）。ケアとホスピタリティは，よいと思われる身体表現を積極的におこなうことで意義が高まる。

Unit 13　Vital Signs

生命徴候

DIALOG　N=nurse,　P=patient

N: Good afternoon, Mr. Davis. How are you feeling today?
P: Pretty good.
N: That's nice. (Checking the oxygen saturation meter) Your oxygen is 96.
P: Great. It was 93 last time, I think.
N: Now, I'd like to take your blood pressure. Let me roll up your sleeve. (Putting a cuff around the patient's upper arm) Please relax. There. Your BP is 140 over 88.
P: It's within my normal range, right?

　N=看護師，P=患者
N: こんにちは、デイヴィスさん。今日のお加減はいかがですか。
P: なかなかいいですよ。
N: よかったですね。(パルスオキシメーターをみて) 酸素は96です。
P: すごいね。前回はたしか93だった。
N: では血圧をはかりましょう。お袖をあげますね。(上腕にカフをまきながら) 力を抜いてください。さあ、終わりました。血圧は140の88です。
P: 私の正常範囲内ですよね。

おぼえておきたい phrases, idioms, grammar

- How are you feeling?
　　Great.「最高にいいです」　Pretty good.「なかなかいいです」　Fine. / OK.「大丈夫です」　Not so good.「あまりよくありません」　Terrible.「とても悪いです」
- What's the matter? / What's the problem?
　　I couldn't sleep well and feel dizzy.

EXERCISE

A． テープを聞いて空所に1語を入れなさい。

N1: How was your weekend?
N2: It was pretty good. I (①   ) camping with my friends.
N1: Oh, really, that (②   ) like fun.
N2: How about you?
N1: On Saturday, I have a night shift. So, on (③   ) I (④   ) to Nikko with my family.
N2: How was the traffic?
N1: Terrible. It took us about 6 hours to get (⑤   ) home.

B． 日本文にあうように（　）内に1語を入れなさい。

1. ヴァイタルサインをしらべましょう。
   I'd (　　　) to take your vital signs.
2. 脈をはかります。
   I'm going to check your (　　　).
3. 腕を出してください。
   Hold (　　　) your arm, please.
4. 深呼吸をしてください。
   Please take a (　　　) breath.
5. 手をしっかり握ってください。
   Please (　　　) a tight fist.

C． テープを聞いて書き取りなさい。

1. (6語) _____

2. (5語) _____

D. テープを聞いて空所をうめましょう。

<Essay 5> Vegetarian Mums 'More Likely To Have Girl Babies'

A vegetarian diet can increase a woman's chances of having a female baby, according to a team of researchers at Nottingham University. They surveyed around 6,000 pregnant (①   ) on the effect of diet on them in 1998 and report that the ratio of male to female births in vegetarians is 85 boys to 100 girls, compared to the national (②   ) of 106 boys born to every 100 girls.

The researchers, who happened on the findings by chance, are at a loss to explain exactly what mechanisms are involved. One (③   ) is that vegetarian women may be put under stress by their diet so that the more robust female fetuses are more likely to (④   ).

The researchers also suggest that a vegetarian (⑤   ) may contain chemicals that mimic the action of female sex hormones such as estrogen.

全訳
＜エッセイ5＞菜食主義のママは『女の赤ちゃんに恵まれる』
　ノッティンガム大学の研究チームによると，菜食主義の食事は，女の赤ちゃんに恵まれる可能性を増やします。彼らは妊娠中の女性にあたえる食事の影響について1998年に約6,000人の妊婦を調査して，菜食主義者から生まれる男女の比率が，全国的な平均値である男106人，女100人に対し，男85人，女100人であると発表しています。
　偶然この結果を見出した研究者達は，それがどういうメカニズムに依るものかを解明できていません。1つの考えは，菜食主義の女性はその食事によりストレスの下に置かれるので，より頑強な女の胎児が生き残りそうであるということです。
　研究者達はまた，菜食主義の食事が，エストロゲンのような女性ホルモンに似た働きをする化学物質を含んでいるかもしれないことを示唆しています。

E. 次の文を日本語にしなさい。
1. A vegetarian diet can increase a woman's chances of having a female baby.

2. The researchers, who happened on the finding by chance, are at a loss to explain exactly what mechanisms are involved.

F. 次の単語の反対語を英語で書きなさい。
1. (　　　　) ⟷ woman
2. boy ⟷ (　　　　)
3. (　　　　) ⟷ female
4. birth ⟷ (　　　　)
5. increase ⟷ (　　　　)

───── How's everything?「お具合はいかがですか」「問題はありませんか」─────

ある入院病棟の看護師長は，気配りや目配りが行き届いている。「看護師はいそがしいですからね」と言って，時間が取れるとこまめに病室をのぞき，患者に声をかけて回っていた。

　"How's everything?" "Is everything all right?" などと気楽に声をかけつつ，実は患者の声の調子や表情を見ているらしい。見舞い客が少なくて内心さびしさを感じている患者，逆に見舞い客が多すぎて安静を保てない患者，だれかれとなく他の病室の患者を訪問する患者など，さまざまな患者がいる。個々の状況に応じた看護を実行することは，はたで考えるほどたやすくないであろうが，プロならではの技術とケアが，さまざまな立場からおこなわれているのは心強い。業務では，ポイントを押さえたことばをさりげなくかける (Spot Conversation：定点会話) 姿勢を大事にしたい。

Unit 14 Rehabilitation

機能回復訓練

DIALOG N＝nurse, P＝patient

N: You look better these days. Let's try to walk slowly today.
P: Well, I don't think I can.
N: I'm sure you can do it. I think you're ready for the training.
P: OK. I'll try.
N: Don't worry. I'll show you how. Like this. Keep your balance.
P: Wow. Thank you. I made it!
N: Keep on practicing. Your muscles will be stronger day by day.

N＝看護師，P＝患者
N: この頃だいぶよくなられたようですね。今日からゆっくりと歩いてみましょう。
P: できるかな。
N: できますよ。もうこの訓練をしていい頃だと思います。
P: じゃ，やってみましょうか。
N: 心配しないでください。やり方をお見せします。こういうふうに。バランスをとって。
P: ふー。ありがとう。できた。
N: 練習を続けてください。筋肉が一日一日回復してきますよ。

おぼえておきたい phrases, idioms, grammar

・励ましの表現
  You're doing well.「調子はいいですよ」 Don't give up.「あきらめないで」
  You did well.「よくがんばりましたね」 You've made it.「よくやりましたね」
・動詞 do＝～を処理する　の使い方
  do the housework, do the dishes, do the laundry, do one's hair, do the gardening

EXERCISE

A. テープを聞いて空所に1語を入れなさい。

F＝patient's family,　N＝nurse

F: He's been (①　　) in bed for weeks. So his arms and legs have been so stiff. How can I help him?

N: Well... Lift his arm gently above his head. Then, slowly (②　　) to the prior position.

F: Like this?

N: Right. Now let's try to move his legs. Flex the (③　　). Then, rotate the foot. Do these exercises 6 or 7 times daily.

B. 日本文にあうように（　）内に1語を入れなさい。

1. 膝をまげましょう。
   (　　　) your knees.
2. 足の裏を床につけてください。
   (　　　) your feet on the floor.
3. 私の手をつかんでください。
   (　　　) my hand.
4. 両腕をぐっと伸ばしてください。
   (　　　) your arms.
5. うつぶせに寝てください。
   (　　　) down (　　　) your stomach.

C. テープを聞いて書き取りなさい。

1. (9語) _____

2. (8語) _____

D. 次の言葉に対する応答の言葉を選びなさい。同じ応答を何度使ってもよい。

1. Here's your hospital gown. ( )
2. I'd like you to meet my partner, Ken. ( )
3. It's my birthday today. ( )
4. You look great in your uniform. ( )
5. See you tomorrow. ( )
6. My dog died last night. ( )
7. I passed the National Examination. ( )
8. Would you like something to drink? ( )
9. I have a terrible headache. ( )
10. Thank you very much for everything. ( )
11. May I come in? ( )
12. I'm sorry. ( )

    a. Nice to meet you.
    b. Congratulations.
    c. Thanks.
    d. Yes, please.
    e. Good-bye.
    f. That's all right.
    g. You're welcome.
    h. I'm sorry to hear that.
    i. Happy birthday.

E. 左の語の意味をあらわすものを右側から選びなさい。
1. recover   (   ) daily meals
2. discharge (   ) schedule for meeting next time
3. diet   (   ) get well
4. exercise   (   ) allow somebody to leave
5. appointment (   ) activity designed for bodily training

F. 空所に適切な疑問詞を入れ，文を完成させなさい。
1. (   ) told you so?
2. (   ) do you have for breakfast?
3. (   ) do you go to school? By bicycle or by bus?
4. (   ) do you have lunch? At home or at school?
5. (   ) do you do your homework? Before or after dinner?

Thank you for saying so.「そうおっしゃっていただき，ありがとうございます」

医療看護の従事者であるからといって，病人や患者に一方的に尽くす立場にあるとばかりは言えない。時には，患者から大いに励まされ助けられていることがある。また患者の一言が，失敗や事故を未然に防ぐのに役立つこともある。

仕事は完璧を目指す…。これは当然の態度だが，思わぬ落とし穴が待ち受けていることもある。病気に立ち向かうためには，患者，家族，担当者が互いに協力し合うことが求められている。

患者およびその家族から，治療や看護に対して「おかしい」「事実を知りたい」「納得いかない」などの疑問や希望，指摘を受けたら，まず事実確認をし，誠意をもって説明しよう。そういった事態に遭遇した時には，"Thank you for saying so."と率直に感謝し，信頼関係を築くチャンスとしたい。

Unit 15 Bed-bath and Positioning

清拭と体位変換

DIALOG　N＝nurse, P＝patient

N: Mr. Davis, I'm going to give you a bed-bath.
P: That sounds nice.
N: First, I'll do your face and neck. ... Now, your arms and chest. ... Then I'll wash your back.
P: Oh, this backrub feels so good.
N: It helps your circulation too.
P: Yes？ That's so relaxing. Thank you.

　　N＝看護師，P＝患者
N: デイヴィスさん，清拭をいたしましょう。
P: いいですね。
N: まず，お顔と首から始めます。…では，腕と胸にいきます。…それでは，お背中を。
P: 背中のマッサージは実に気持ちがいいですね。
N: 血液の循環にもいいのですよ。
P: そう？ほんとうに楽になった。ありがとう。

おぼえておきたい phrases, idioms, grammar

・意向を聞かれた場合の応答
　Shall I open the window？
　　　（肯定）Yes, please.
　　　（否定）No, thank you.
　Would you like tea or coffee？
　　　（I'd like）tea, please. または Coffee, please.

EXERCISE

A. テープを聞いて空所に1語を入れなさい。

N: You need to change your position (①   ) few hours to prevent a bedsore or pneumonia.

P: It hurts to move.

N: Please take a deep (②   ) and slowly breathe out. ... Now, (③   ) me pull your pajama top. I'll put one pillow under your left leg and another one (④   ) your back.

P: I'm (⑤   ) more comfortable. Thank you.

B. 日本文にあうように（　）内に1語を入れなさい。

1. シャンプーをしましょうか。
   Would you (   ) a shampoo?
2. 足を洗います。
   I'm going to wash your (   ).
3. 包帯をぬらさないようにしてください。
   Please (   ) your bandage dry.
4. おしもはご自分で洗われますか。
   Could you wash your private parts by (   )?
5. 手助けが必要な時はいってください。
   Please let me (   ) if you need any help.

C. テープを聞いて書き取りなさい。

1. (6語) _____

2. (7語) _____

D. 次の文の間違いを直しなさい。

例：What your name ? → What's your name ?

1. How do you feeling ?
   → _____

2. I'm very interesting in nursing.
   → _____

3. What do you say "*jinzo*" in English ?
   → _____

4. Where are you come from ?
   → _____

5. My grandfather was died last year.
   → _____

6. What's she doing ? She checks the patient's urine sample.
   → _____

Call me at any time.「いつでもお呼びください」「ご用の際はお声をかけてください」

　病院もホスピタリティ産業の1つとされる。患者サービスは，十分に実行されているであろうか。
　「よい品を安く」というのは消費者の願いだが，病院は「よい品（技術・環境など）は高い」と提示しても，病人にボイコットされることはない。それだけに，無駄な治療はしないなど，患者の立場に立ったサービスの徹底が望まれる。"Call me at any time."の応対サービスは，その1つであろう。
　経済活動の一環として実施されるサービスは，品質・値段・環境などの諸条件が上乗せされ，サービス料金となって値段が表示される。ホスピタリティは料金提示はされない。行為を実施する者も，受ける者も，互いに満たされる気持ちになるのが特徴といえる。清潔な服装や化粧，機敏な立ち居ふるまいや物言い，声の強弱，語彙力など，ホスピタリティの実行者は，言語・非言語コミュニケーション技能と感性の涵養を視野に入れる必要があるであろう。We are what we speak and do.（話すこととすることで人がわかる）

付録　総復習すごろくゲーム

グループですごろくをしよう。サイコロの目だけ進み，その問いに答えなさい。

START					
Where do you come from?	Could I borrow your eraser?	Who do you live with?	What do you do in your free time?	How do you spell your name?	

- How do you say "Hello" in Korean?
- How do you say "Thank you" in Portuguese?
- Say these numbers: 1,200 / 12,000 / 120,000 / 1,200,000
- Tell me about your family.
- How do you feel today?
- Excuse me, where's the restroom?
- Lucky! Go forward one space.
- Tell me five parts of the body.
- Have you ever had any serious illnesses?
- Have you ever traveled abroad?
- What are you studying?
- How long have you been studying in this school?
- What did you do last weekend?
- What will you be doing in 10 years?
- Sorry! Go back 1 space.
- Tell me 3 medical departments in English.
- Do you mind if I smoke?
- Would you do me a favor?
- Tell me about your class teacher.
- What are you going to do during your next vacation?
- Where is the nearest station?
- How often do you work at a part-time job?
- Will you be a nurse with care and hospitality?
- FINISH

ケアとホスピタリティの英語 Ⅰ

著　者　　古閑　博美／垂石　幸与／土谷　宣子

2001年4月1月　第1刷発行
2020年4月1日　第5刷発行

発行者　寺内由美子
発行所　鷹書房弓プレス
　　　　〒162-0802　東京都新宿区改代町33-17
　　　　電話　03(5261)8470　FAX　03(5261)8474
　　　　振替　00100-2-148033

ISBN978-4-8034-1215-4　C 1082